Surviving Myself

Wounds That Speak, Words That Heal

By

DeJuana Edwards

Published by DeJuanaCreativeHoldings LLC
First Edition: 2025
ISBN: 979-8-218-68159-3

This book is a work of creative nonfiction. The experiences,
reflections, and expressions within are the author's truth, shaped by
lived experiences and poetic interpretation.

For permission or inquiries, contact:
dejuana@dejuanacreative.com

Printed in the United States of America.

To the loved ones I carry in my heart—
Your memory lives in every word.

To those still fighting—
May these pages remind you that you are
never alone

To the version of me that kept going—
I'm proud of you for staying.

Epigraph

*"In the depths of my soul, where pain and healing
intertwine poetry became my voice"*

—DeJuana Edwards

Trigger Warning: Disclaimer

This book contains honest reflections and raw expression of real-life emotions including experiences with depression, anxiety, trauma, and suicidal thoughts. These words are not meant to glorify, condone, influence, or promote suicide in any way, form, or fashion.

Surviving Myself: Wounds That Speak, Words That Heal is my truth—a testimony to the darkness I've lived through and the healing I'm still learning. My intention is not to harm, but to speak what is often silenced, to let others know they're not alone, and to remind anyone reading: there is help, there is hope, and your life matters.

If you are struggling, please know you are not alone. Reach out. Speak up. There is no shame in needing support.

National Suicide & Crisis Lifeline (US):988
Crisis Text Line: Text Home to 741741

Letter to Reader

Dear Reader,

Before you turn the page, I want to say—thank you.
Thank you for picking up this book, for being curious, for being
open, and most importantly, for showing up.

Surviving Myself: Wounds That Speak, Words That Heal is not
just a collection of poems—it's a part of me. Every word you'll
read was born from a place of pain, growth, healing, and truth. This
book is my testimony. My breaking. My becoming.

I've walked through the silence of depression, battled the shadows
of anxiety, and stood face-to-face with thoughts I never thought I'd
speak out loud. But I'm still here—and if you're reading this so are
you.

This book isn't here to fix you. It's not a manual or solution. It is a
mirror. A hug. A whisper in the dark that says, "You are not
alone". It is proof that wounds can speak—and when they do, they
can also help heal others.

Whether you are in the middle of your own storm or simply
seeking to understand someone else's, I hope these pages meet you
where you are. Let them hold space for your heart, your tears, your
questions, and your healing.

You'll notice there's no table of contents. That's intentional.
Healing isn't linear, and neither is this book. Life didn't hand me a
map through my pain, so I won't hand you one either. Let these
words find you as they may.

With love and light,
DeJuana Edwards

Foreword

It takes incredible courage to give voice to the battles we often fight in silence. This book of poetry shares a powerful journey through darkness, healing, and growth. Each poem stands as a testament to resilience—a reminder that even in our hardest moments, there is strength in vulnerability and power in honesty.

By choosing to speak up, you have not only claimed your own light but also offered hope to others still searching for theirs.

Congratulations on these beautiful and brave accomplishments. Your words will reach the hearts that need them most.

—Precious B.

Acknowledgments

First and foremost, I want to thank God—for His grace, mercy, and for keeping me when I didn't want to be kept. Through the darkest nights and the heaviest storms, He never let go of me.

To my beautiful children: Rashad, Rodreyonna, Rai Juan—you are my heartbeat, my light, my reason. Your existence reminds me every day why I must keep fighting. I love you more than words can ever say.

Precious—my best friend, my sister in spirit, you've walked with me through my darkest valleys, picked me up when I couldn't stand, poured into me when I was empty, and loved me without judgement. Our friendship has healed me in ways I can never repay, and it means the world to me.

Kayla K—my best friend, my longest friend, over a decade of love, laughter, and loyalty. You've been there without fail, helped care for my children, and stood by me through everything. We're more like family than friends. Friendmily. I'm endlessly grateful for you.

Arron—thank you for the words of affirmations, the protection, the shoulders to cry on, and the encouragement you've poured into me over the years. You've reminded me of my strength and the power of my story.

Kay—AKA Sistuhhhhhh, even though you're the newest in my life, it feels like we've known each other forever. You've gone above and beyond, always uplifting me with love and understanding. We call each other sisters, and we truly are. Two peas in a pod.

My brother DeJuan—I love you more than words can describe. Your support, your loyalty, your belief in me…I don't know what I would do without you. You've always had my back, always rooted for me. I couldn't have asked for a better big brother. I love you.

Lastly, I honor the memory of my cousin, Keysue Boone and my dear friend, Dexter Sims, whose lives were lost to suicide. Your pain birthed my purpose, and I will carry your names with me always. This book is for you. This journey is because of you.

To everyone who stood by me, believed in me, and loved me through my pain and healing—this book is a piece of my soul, and it exists because of you. Thank you.

Introduction

Green is more than just a color—it's the international symbol for mental health awareness.

Green represent mental health because it signifies hope, growth, and renewal. It is a reminder of healing and life.

Green symbolizes breaking the silence, understanding, and creating a safe space for open conversations.

I Should've Been Left There

"I should've left your ass there—bleeding"
Words not just spoken, but seething.
Dripping venom in a moment of rage
Etched on my soul like ink on this page.

I still see that floor, still feel that night.
When I almost lost the will to fight
A slit wrist and silent scream—
My life unraveling in a broken dream.

And she found me—shook me back.
A lifeline in the darkest black
But months would pass and words would
fly
And in that fight, she let truth die.

Because even in anger, even in pain
There are things you don't say, things that
stain
But she said it, sharp and cold.
A bullet of betrayal, brutal and bold

I should've been gone, that's what she
meant
Like I was a burden, like my life was spent.
Like my bleeding body didn't deserve care
Just to be left lifeless, gasping for air

But let me tell you what those words did.
They found the fire I thought I'd hid.
They struck a match inside my soul.
And made my broken pieces whole.

Because if I survived that kind of hate
Then maybe I wasn't meant for fate.
That ends in silence, pain, and gloom.

Maybe I'm here to light up the room.

Maybe I'm here to speak out loud.
To rise above, to make her proud
Not her, the friend who walked away.
But the me I lost that fatal day

The me who thought that death was peace.
That ending it all would bring release.
But now I see I am the proof.
That life goes on past pain and truth.

That healing hurts but so does hate.
And sometimes people show you fate.
Not by lifting but by throwing knives.
And still, you rise and save your life.

Now I wake with a different fire.
Fueled not by vengeance but something
Higher
To show the world I didn't die.
To look depression in the eye

To tell anxiety, "You don't own me."
To tell those dark thoughts, "Set me free."
Because someone said I should be gone
But I'm still here still holding on.

And every breath I take is proof.
That I can stand inside my truth
So, say what you want, think what you will.
But I'm still breathing, I'm here still.

And for anyone who's heard those words
Like knives disguised in mockingbirds
Let this be your battle cry.
You lived, you rose, you didn't die.

Because sometimes hate's the spark you
need
To plant your roots and stop the bleed.
Sometimes the cruelest things they say.
Can push your darkest thoughts away.

So, no, I wasn't left to die.
And now I live, I speak, I try.
This is my truth, my war, my art.
And healing started with a broken heart.

Still Here

To the one reading this with heavy eyes
Who's mastered the art of silent cries.
Who smiles in crowds but breaks alone—
I see you; I know that tone.

You've danced with demons in your mind.
Fought thoughts that weren't so kind.
You've begged the night to end your ache.
And wondered how much more you'd take.

But guess what? You're still here.
Breathing, hurting, wiping the tears.
And that my friend, is no small feat—
That's courage standing on its feet.

Depression lies, says you're too weak.
That hope is gone, that life's too bleak
But every time you've faced the storm.
You didn't shatter—you transformed.

Anxiety may steal your air.
Make you feel trapped and unaware.
But you keep going, step by step.
Even shaking, you always kept

And those thoughts that scream.
That life's too much, that peace is a
dream—
Let me tell you something true:
The world is better because of you.

You have a heart that's felt too much.
A soul that longs for gentle touch
You love so deep it leaves you raw—
That's not weakness, that's your core

You are not broken, you're a flame.
A warrior with a sacred name
And if todays' too much to bear
Just know there's strength in being there.

Loving yourself might feel so far.
But healing starts right where you are.
Not in perfection, not in speed—
But in each breath, in every need

So, hold on, even when it's rough.
Even when you feel not enough.
There's light in you the dark can't kill.
A fire that flickers, burning still.

And when the world says, "You can't rise."
Look in the mirror, defy those lies.
Say, "I'm still here, I've come this far—
My battle scars are who I am."

You are proof that pain survives.
But never owns or steals our lives.
You're strength and fire, love and grace—
And this world needs your sacred place.

So, stay. Breathe. Begin again.
The story's yours—not when it ends.
You've got power, soul, and voice.
To fight back hard—and make the choice.

To live. To heal. To rise above.
To choose yourself. To choose self-love.

The Urge

Alone and drowned in darkness.
Mind telling you to do it.
Mentally unstable? I already knew it.
Mind playing tricks.
Devil in your ear
Death by suicide, decision seems so clear.

Constant battles within self
I wish there was more light shed on mental
health
I am not okay; this I can admit.
Death by suicide just makes sense.

Drowned in depression, anxiety, and stress
too
Look me in my eyes and tell me what would
you do
Trying to hold on and fight back the urge.
I am the target, myself I purge.

Thinking of ways to end this for good
Never say I won't when I know
I probably would

The Silence I Broke

I've buried pain beneath my smile.
Carried grief in every mile.
Lost two souls I loved so dear.
To silence, sorrow, shame, and fear.

A cousin's laugh, a friend's warm light
Now flicker starts in endless night.
They left too soon; their battles lost.
And I'm left counting every cost.

It's different—this type of goodbye.
It whispers why with no reply.
You don't just mourn, you question fate.
And wonder why you saw too late

Was there a sign I failed to see?
A message lost inside of me?
When your own mind is breaking too
It's hard to notice pain in view.

You send a text, but not in vain—
You know no answers coming again.
That void, that echo, hits so deep
It keeps you up when you should sleep.

But through the tears, I found a flame.
A softer strength inside the pain
Their deaths, a wound I'll always bear.
But now I fight with louder care.

I couldn't save them, that is true—
But I can try to heal for you.
For anyone who's felt the fall
Who hides their truth behind a wall?

I've wanted out, I've felt that break.

The weight too much for me to take
But something in me chose to stay.
To turn my night into a day

I speak now, not for me alone.
But for the hearts that feel unknown
I've tasted loss in suicide's name.
But from that loss, I rise in flame.

Because I know that kind of hurt
The kind that makes your soul feel dirt
But I won't let it steal my voice—
Survival now is my loud choice.

How strange the way pain makes you grow.
Like flowers blooming under snow
So weak, so strong, both sides I show—
I break, I rise, I learn, I grow.

I share my scars to light the way.
For those still fighting through the gray
And if my truth can spare one soul
Then breaking silence makes me whole.

The Other Side of Depression

Depression isn't always
Tears streaming down a tired face.
In the middle of the night
With the lights off and the curtains drawn

Sometimes—
It's laughter that doesn't reach the soul.
Smiles stretched too wide.
Jokes told just loud enough, to drown out the ache.

It's showing up.
Even when every bone begs you to stay home
It's being the light in the room.
While your own world is flickering dim

It's "I'm okay"
Said with a grin.
Because explaining the fog
Feels heavier than the fog itself.

Sometimes depression looks like productivity.
Checking every box on the list
Because the silence is too deafening
When you stop

It wears makeup, and post selfies.
Answer, "How are you?"
With, "I'm good"
Because who would believe otherwise?

It isn't always lying in bed for days.
Sometimes it's being surrounded by people
And still feeling
Completely alone

Sometimes, depression wears bright colors.

And it still feels gray inside.
It holds space in hearts.
You'd least expect.

So be gentle.
With the ones who shine the most
They might be using their light
To find their own way home

Try What Heals You

When the weight feels too heavy to carry
And your soul forgets how to rise.
Know that healing isn't a finish line.
It's a series of small tries.

Try therapy.
Let the words fall out like rain.
Let someone sit with your silence.
Hold your pain without judgement.

Try picking up something new
A brush, a pen, a plant, a puzzle
Let your hands remember the joy
Your heart forgot.

Try walking, even if it's slow.
Even if it's just to the mailbox and back.
Let your body move toward the light.
One step at a time

Try prayer.
Whisper it or weep it.
To God, the universe, or your own heart
Let hope echo in the quiet

Try doing what use to bring you peace.
Music, baking, dancing alone in your room
Joy doesn't have to be loud to be real.

Try resting.
Not because you're lazy.
But because surviving is exhausting
And you deserve softness, too.

Try talking to a friend.
Or writing to yourself

Or screaming into a pillow
Just to hear your voice again

Try grace.
Over and over and over
Especially on the days
When getting up feels impossible

You don't have to do it all.
Just try what heals you, piece by piece
Breath by breath
You're worth the effort it takes to keep going.

From Wounds to Wings

They told me to hush.
To bury the ache
To smile through storms
My soul couldn't fake.

But silence is heavy.
And pain doesn't sleep.
It carves out a corner
In the places you keep

I wore my wounds.
Like invisible thread
Stitched into stones
I never had said.

Until one day
I picked up a pen
And wrote down the fire
That burned deep within

Each word was a mirror.
Each line a release
Each poem a prayer
For a moment of peace

I turned all the trauma
They told me to hide.
Into something that lives
Something that rides.

I turned shame into strength.
Grief into grace
Fear into flames.
That lit up my space.

This book is my offering.

My battle- scarred truth
A voice for the hurting
The silenced, the youth

It's proof you can fall
And still find your rise
That power lives quiet
In tear- stained eyes

So here I stand.
No longer concealed.
A wound that speaks.
A word that heals.

Pulse

Suicide I contemplate daily.
Will I ever go through with it? One day, maybe
I'm tired of fighting, I feel so alone.
Might as well say fuck it, call myself home.

Mentally unstable, it's hard to fight back.
It's something inside of me, something I lack.
Childhood trauma, adult trauma too
Point me in the right direction, I don't know what to do.

Depression eats me up inside and out.
Feels like death is the only way out.
I cry as I write this, "How is this my life?"
I'm a good person, why so much strife?

I walk around smiling like I am okay.
Truth be told, I want to die every day.
My head fucked up and my hearts up for sale.
My whole life turned upside down when I went to jail.

My soul full of pain, all I want is peace
God, can you please let up some, at least?
I battle between living and dying.
I am so fucking tired of crying.

My thoughts are my worst enemies.
And my demons come out to play.
Just one bullet
Will take it all away.

Stop minimizing mental health, this shit is real.
I'll never forget my temple against that steel.
Cutting and digging, fucking up my flesh
Lay down, never wake up, I think that's best.

Can't talk to my brother.

Can't talk to my mom.
Crazy
I use to depend on the 23rd Psalm.

In a world so cold
I'm convinced.
I'm just existing.
Numerous suicide attempts—just failed at my mission.

I try to stay positive.
Try to stay strong.
God, what did I do?
That was so fucking wrong.

Living in my own misery
I don't know how I deal.
It's this thing called a pulse.
That I just want to kill

One word I think of
When it comes to me
Hate
Answer me this, can death really wait?

Those that know, know.
Most won't understand.
I'm trying my best to instead.
Wait for God's plan.

To understand this piece
Read between the lines
As I let this pen cease

I Am Not My Past

I've done things I don't talk about
Wore guilt like skin, stitched in doubt.
But I am more than where I've been.
More than shame I carried within

I'm growth and grit, I'm rising fast.
My name is not tied to my past.
I'm not what broke me, not what I lacked.
I'm the comeback they never tracked.

I've worn mistakes like second skin.
Let guilt take root and grow within
I've replayed moments, a thousand times.
Where silence screamed and healing hid in rhymes

I've walked through rooms with my head hung low.
Thinking everyone saw what I didn't show.
I've begged for grace I thought I didn't deserve.
Punished myself with every swerve.

I've been judged by chapters they never read.
Defined by rumors, by what they said.
But let me be clear, let me make it last.
I am not my wounds; I am not my past.

I am not the nights I cried alone.
Or the brokenness I tried to atone.
Not the hands that hurt the bridges burned
Or all the lessons I had to learn.

I am the fire that wouldn't fade.
The strength that sorrow could never invade.
I am the fight beneath the tears.
The voice that rose above my fears

Yes, I've fallen again and again.

But each time, I stood, each time I began.
Not polished, not perfect, and free from the scars
But proud of how I've made it this far.

I am the story they thought would end.
The silence that chose to speak again
I am growth wrapped in broken truth.
A living poem, a resilient proof

So, don't you dare define me still
By who I was when I lacked will
By what I did when I couldn't see
The light that lived inside of me

Because now I rise with purpose clear
A different voice, a different year
Not bound by shame, nor tethered fast.
I am not my pain; I am not my past.

Healing Isn't Pretty

Healing isn't roses or warm sunlight.
It's shaking hands in the middle of the night.
It's tears on a pillow then doing it again.
It's one step forward, then back where you've been.

It's not always peace, or clean- cut lines.
It's reliving moments that shattered time.
But messy or not, each scar I see.
Is proof that healing still chose me

It's ugly crying in a bathroom stall.
It's isolation when you can't make a call.
It's doubting progress, it's starting slow.
It's wondering if you'll ever let go.

It's journaling thoughts you're scared to read.
It's feeling hollow and full of need.
It's choosing life in a quiet fight.
Even when you don't sleep at night.

It's breaking cycles that felt like home.
Undoing lies you've always known.
It's facing truths that feel like flames.
Then rising up and naming names

It's praying when you don't believe.
And hoping without guarantees
It's forgiving yourself, piece by piece.
It's holding on until there's peace.

It's not sunrise every day.
Sometimes it's just finding the will to stay.
It's not a quote, or a perfect scene.
It's a messy, real, and in- between

But in that mess, there lives your light.

The proof you're still putting up a fight.
You're not broke; you're becoming free.
Because healing, my love, isn't pretty, it's brave. It's me.

Dear Younger Me

Dear younger me, the one with tired eyes
The one who learned too soon how the world lies.
Who smiled in pain and laughed to cope.
Who held on tight to slivers of hope.

You didn't deserve the weight you bore.
The silence behind every closed door
You should've been dancing, chasing the sun.
Not wondering if you were ever the one.

You thought love was something you had to earn.
That worth was tied to every turn.
But you were magic even then.
A masterpiece before, not after, the mend

You didn't need to shrink to fit.
To bury your light or silence your wit.
You were never too loud or too deep.
You just needed a safe place to weep.

You did what you could with what you knew.
And somehow still, you always grew.
So, don't regret how you survived.
You gave your all just to stay alive.

I wish someone had told you then.
You are not your trauma, not where you've been.
You're not your scars, your pain, your fears.
You're so much more than your hidden tears.

It's okay you didn't always speak.
That you had days when you were weak
You were learning strength in quiet ways.
Becoming fire in your own blaze

So, if you're still carrying shame or doubt.

Let's start the healing from inside out.
You were always worthy, don't forget.
Even when life hadn't shown you yet.

The dreams you held. They're still alive.
The parts of you lost. You will revive.
You'll learn to love the skin you're in
To stand back up and fight again.

You'll cry. You'll break. You'll question why.
But you'll also soar and touch the sky.
And one day when your finally free
You'll look back proud and say, "Look what I've done for me."

Give Yourself Grace

They say, be strong.
But never taught me what to do when strength runs dry
When silence screams louder than words
And the mirror reflects a stranger's eyes.

I've walked through storms dressed in smiles
Hid behind, "I'm fine", while drowning in noise
It's messy, raw, and real.
A testimony whispered between the cracks of broken days.

It's okay to not be okay
To fall apart, to shatter under the weight of invisible battles
Your scars don't make you weak.
They tell the story of how you stayed.

I've stitched poems from pain.
Turned wounds into words that bleed light.
Each verse a confession
Each stanza, a breath I thought I'd never take.

And in chaos, I've learned this truth.
Healing doesn't mean you're always whole.
Even when the world forgets your name.
Don't forget your worth.

Give yourself grace on the days you can't get out of bed.
When your heart is too heavy to carry
When all you can do is breathe
You are not a failure for feeling.

You are human.
You are hurting.
You are healing.
And that, in itself, is enough.

The Weight Didn't Win

I've walked through shadows, cold and deep.
Silent battles, nights with no sleep
A heart that ached, a mind that screamed
A soul once lost in shattered dreams.

But here I stand—a living sign.
Proof that pain won't steal my shine.
The weight was heavy, the road was rough.
Yet, I refused to say, "Enough."

I've danced with darkness, faced the fall.
But I found my voice and broke the wall.
Now my story spills like ink on pages
A fight for hope through all life's stages

For those still trapped in silent cries
Know the sun still waits to rise
You're not alone, your heart still beats.
There's light ahead in every piece.

Afterword: The Stone Rolled Away

If Jesus got out of the grave
Then I can get out of depression
Because the resurrection didn't stop at Calvary
It continues in me.

In every breath I didn't think I'd take
In every tear I thought would drown me
In every night I made it through when the weight felt too heavy
Hope didn't die. It rose.

This book is my resurrection, my silent screams turned to spoken truth.
My wounds-once hidden- now speak healing.
Every poem, every page, is proof.
That darkness doesn't get the final say.

I am a walking testimony.
Not because I never broke.
But because I refused
To stay buried

So, if you're reading this and you are still in your valley.
Still wrestling with shadows, remember this:
You're not alone, you're beyond saving.
You are worthy of life-full life.

Let this be your sign, your light, your reminder:
If He got up, you can get up too.
And when you do, don't just survive. Rise.

Not Just a Hashtag

Everybody wants to be an expert now.
Quoting things, they don't even know how.
But if you haven't lived it, don't speak on my pain.
You can't preach healing if you've never felt rain.

You talk about suicide like it's just a word.
But behind that word are voices unheard
You shame the anxious, mock the depressed.
But never once asked why they're stressed.

You judge what you see, but not what is true.
That smile they wear might be hiding a bruise.
So quick to be cruel, so fast to condemn.
But what if tomorrow, it's you or it's them?

Stop being nasty, stop being blind.
You don't know the war in somebody's mind.
That weird kid? That "too quiet" friend?
Might be holding on by a fragile end.

If you really cared, you'd choose your words.
Speak life instead of throwing swords.
Love a little louder, ask twice to stay near.
Be the light when the dark feels near

Mental health isn't some online trend.
Its real life battles that people defend.
So, show up with kindness, lead with your heart.
Change doesn't happen unless you start.

Smile at strangers, offer your time.
Say, "I'm here" and truly mean the line.
This world could heal if we just believed.
That being human means all souls grieve.

So, love more deeply.

And judge way less
Because compassion is
How we heal this mess

Green Means Go

Green is the color of starting again.
Of healing the heart, of paper, and pen
It's a growth in the cracks where the light softly glows.
A symbol of strength only silence knows.

In May we wear it—this ribbon, this hue
For battles fought daily that no one sees through.
Not broke, but bending still choosing to fight.
Still chasing the sun in the darkest of night

It's not always pretty this path that we take.
Some days were just breathing, just trying not to break.
But green means you're growing, no matter the pace.
And every small win deserves gentle grace.

It's therapy sessions and tears on the floor.
It's journaling pain you can't speak anymore.
It's praying for peace when your spirit feels low.
It's showing up still—when you'd rather not go.

It's doing the work they may never applaud.
It's crying to music; it's talking to God.
It's dancing alone just to feel something true.
It's choosing yourself when the world isn't you

It's saying, "no" softly, to protect your own peace.
It's resting without needing reasons or release.
It's finding the courage to voice what you've faced.
And building a life you don't need to fake.

May is for truth, for breaking the shame.
For saying out loud, "I'm not playing the game."
Mental health matters, it's not just a trend.
It's loving yourself like your own dearest friend.

So, this May let the color remind you, your seen.

That hope isn't lost, and healing is green,
You're not just surviving, you're learning to grow.
And every step forward is green, saying: Go.

Fight Back

I used to think silence was strong.
That not speaking meant I could carry on.
That hiding pain made me brave and wise.
That holding it in meant I'd survive.

But I had it wrong, so wrong I see.
Silence was a case that imprisoned me.
It wasn't strength to fake the light.
While I was drowning deep at night

Now I challenge you, whoever you are.
With hidden scars and a shattered heart
Don't let silence steal your name.
Don't bow your head, don't play that game.

Fight back with every breath you take.
With every tear with every break
Fight back when it whispers, "You're not enough."
When life gets cruel, and days get tough.

Speak even if your voice shakes loudly.
Cry, even if they disappear or crowd.
You are not weak for needing space.
You are not broken for craving grace.

Fight back against the weight you hide.
Against the thoughts that say you shouldn't try
You are worthy of the fight you give.
You are proof that hurt can live, and still be healed, and still
forgive.

You are not the ending in your head.
You are not better off silent or dead.
You are here. You are light. You are breathing.
And that alone has already cheated death

So, scream if you must. Write it down.
Dance in pain. Don't let it drown.
Tell your story—don't you dare forget.
Your survival is your loudest threat.

Lies They Told Us

They said,
"People who smile can't be suicidal."
But baby I was dying with dimples.
Laughing out loud while losing myself quietly
Smiles don't mean safety.
Sometimes they're just armor.

They said,
"You're just being dramatic."
But you weren't there at 3am
When my thoughts turned into thunder
And my heart begged for peace.
In a world that never lets me rest
Drama? Nah. That was desperation

They said,
"Talking about it is attention seeking."
But silence nearly killed me.
I spoke because I wanted to live.
I broke the hush so someone else might hold on.
Truth isn't begging for eyes.
It's building bridges for souls.

They said,
"You have nothing to be sad about."
As if pain sends a warning.
As if trauma checks your bank account.
Nah, sometimes it shows up in the middle of blessings.
And buries you anyway.

They said,
"Stop making excuses."
But this isn't an excuse, this is exhaustion.
This is years of pretending.
This is trying, every day, to stay.
You don't see the battle.

But I fight it anyway.

So, here's the truth:
Mental health isn't a vibe.
It isn't a moment.
It's a lifetime of learning how to breathe.
How to believe, how to be

And if all you've got is judgement, keep it.
Because we're not weak
We're warriors learning how to heal.
In a world that still thinks pain should whisper

Me Vs Me

Childhood trauma led to adult depression.
It's time to break the silence.
Help someone in need through my confessions.

See, a lot of things we experienced as a kid.
Continue to haunt us—daily.
A lot of things done that people don't know.
That were did, quietly, painfully, gravely.

Falling asleep in class, no sleep
The night before, had to keep my eyes open, stay alert
Listening for a twist and turn on a locked door.

Feeling unloved so I turned to the streets.
But you better be careful—
Life's a bitch
Never know who you're going to meet.

Sixteen, moving off emotions with a heart full of rage.
I found myself in a situation.
I couldn't have imagined.
Pregnant, lost.
With the father nearly three times my age

Looking for love in all the wrong places
Will leave you in fucked up situations.
You know what invading personal space is?
Pistol to my head, slices in my skin—
Some call it fighting demons, some let the devil in

I could go on for days, on for nights.
Been crying the same tears for years.
Hold on, embrace yourself.
This poem is about to switch gears.

Sleeping days away, laying in the dark

Turned my emotions and feelings into words—
This pen to this paper is how I start.

Days without washing my ass.
 Body glued to the bed, set suicide to the side.
And wrote this poetry book instead.

Crying, sad, alone, and feeling abandoned
Why do I struggle with mental health?
So much God? Huh?
I'm not understanding.

Shutting down from the world
Phone on DND
Never take it personal
Right now, it's Me Vs Me

Tend to the kids.
Work, clean, cook—
Ask me how I got through the day.
Ask me what it took.

Read, paint, write, run, walk.
Because I know what it's like
To have listen, but no talk

And it doesn't stop there.
The list goes on.
Suicide feels so right.
But I know it's so wrong.

Yes, it's a constant battle.
I know you're tired of hearing "stay strong."
I'm a walking testimony, friend.
I pray you hold on.

So, stop, breathe.
And please think things through

Suicide is a permanent decision.
That can only be decided through you.

If I could make it through, then so can you.
I've cried in silence, felt broken in two.
But somehow, I'm standing—so you can too.

Remember To….

Before you close this final page
Before you walk beyond this stage
Let one truth echo, soft and clear.
Give yourself grace while you're still here.

Not just when you rise and shine.
But when you're lost, unsure, out of line.
Not just when the healing shows
But when it hurts, and no one knows.

Give grace to the one who stayed alive.
Who fought through storms just to survive
The one who cried but still pressed through.
Who made it here—yes, that's you.

Grace for the versions of you that fell.
For the secrets you carried, the pain you won't tell.
For every setback, every slow pace
You deserve love in every place.

This journey was never meant to be perfect, polished, or pain-free.
It was meant to shape your soul with light.
Even when all you did was fight.

So, take a breath, unclench your hands
Forgive yourself—make no demands
Healing takes time, and peace takes space.
Above all else, give yourself grace.

You're not behind: You're not too late.
You're not defined by hurt or fate.
You are becoming, day by day.
Exactly enough, in every way

And when you doubt, when you feel misplaced.
Return to this moment.

And give yourself grace.

Bonus Poem for the Black Man Who Feels Invisible
(A message of love, truth, and affirmations)

Black men,
I'm writing this for you.
I know you say your mental health doesn't matter.
But I promise you it do.

You walk through a world
That often doesn't see you, hear you, or check on your heart.
But I see you, and your loved.
Even if no one's ever told you that part.

It's okay to not be okay
It's okay to cry.
It's okay to say, "I need help."
Because nothing beats a failure but a try

Mental health takes time.
Takes effort, takes grace.
So, if I check in on you, don't push me away.
Don't disappear without a trace.

No, I'll never know what it's like
To live life as a Black man
But I'm standing beside you.
Doing what I can

Being vulnerable doesn't make you weak.
Being vulnerable makes you human.
Do you really feel no one care—
Or are you just assuming?

You are appreciated.
You are wanted.
You are needed.
Chin up, Chest out
A king is never defeated.

If ever your low, revisit this page.
For strength, for love, for truth
I wrote on your behalf this day.

Your worth is not measured by money.
Or what you provide.
Your value is rooted.
In the light you carry inside

You are allowed to feel.
To speak.
To rest.
To just be.

You are seen.
You are worthy.
And you matter—
Deeply

Closing Note

Depression doesn't always look like what you think. It isn't always tears, darkness, or isolation. Sometimes, it wears the mask of laughter, a bright smile, drinking, smoking, over-eating, casual sex—it shows up in ways the world doesn't always recognize.

Mental health doesn't discriminate. It affects people of all ages, races, and backgrounds. Being open, honest, and transparent about our struggles is one of the hardest things to do. Sometimes, it's fear—fear of judgement, fear of being laughed at, not being taken seriously, or just feeling like no one truly cares.

But I'm here to tell you: YOU ARE NOT ALONE

Check on your family, friends, and loved ones. And please—don't forget your strong friend. Oftentimes, it's the strongest ones who are carrying the heaviest burdens and silently fighting battles no one knows about.

Tell someone you love them. Tell someone you care. A single word, small gesture, or being kind can save a life.

This book has been my way of breaking the silence, telling the truth, and creating a safe space for anyone who's ever felt alone in their pain.

Thank you for allowing me to share my story with you. I hope, wherever you are, you are in your journey and that you remember this:

Your life matters. Your voice matters. You matter.

About the Author

At 31, DeJuana Edwards is a survivor, writer, and mental health advocate who uses poetry to transform pain into purpose. Through raw honesty and vulnerability, she shares her personal journey with depression, anxiety, suicidal thoughts, and healing to remind others they are not alone. Her words are more than poetry, they are a testimony of survival. When she's not writing, DeJuana finds peace in music, being near the water, and staying active at the gym. She enjoys spending quality time with her children and loved ones, exploring new foods, and traveling. Above all, she finds joy in helping others—believing that making others smile is one of the greatest gifts of all.

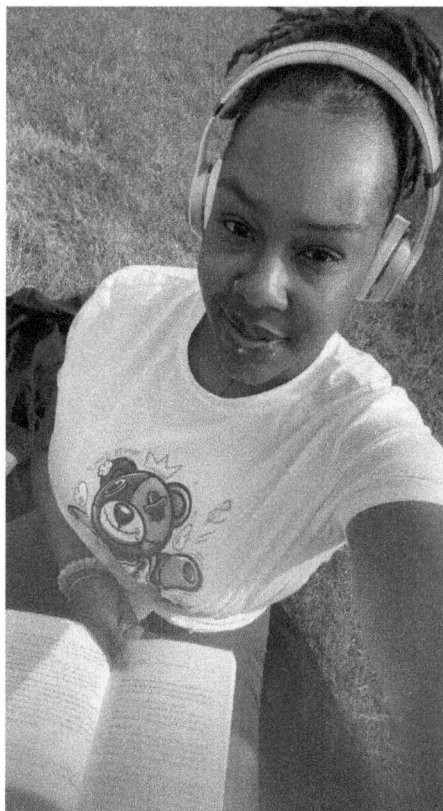

Other Books

Surviving Myself: Wounds That Speak, Words That Heal is my first published book, but it will not be my last. I am already working on future projects that continue to shine a light on the importance of mental health, healing, resilience, and the power of storytelling.

Please stay connected and be on the lookout for upcoming poetry collections, personal reflections, and new releases that will dive even deeper into the journey of survival, growth, and transformation.

Thank you for supporting my voice. Thank you for walking this journey with me.

You haven't seen the last of me—the best is still on its way.

Resources

If you are struggling, you are not alone. Please reach out to one of these sources:

National Suicide Prevention Lifeline
Phone: 988
Website: www.988lifeline.org

Crisis Text Line
Text: HOME to 741741
Website: www.crisistextline.org

National Alliance on Mental Illness (NAMI)
Phone: 1-800-950-NAMI (6264)
Website: www.nami.org

Connect with the Author

Email: dejuana@dejuanacreative.com
Phone: 313-380-1522
Website: www.dejuanacreative.com (COMING SOON!)
Social media: Tiktok @Juana_melaninmonroe|Instagram @Juana_mha

For support, questions, or to share your story—don't hesitate to reach out. You're not alone.